INTRODUCTION

You go to the doctor routinely to preserve your wellness. That's absolutely smart. Before your following consultation, however, consider this: when was the last time your doctor asked about your diet?

Although physicians are perfectly aware of the connection in between our health and wellness as well as the food we took into our body, this is a concern they hardly ever, if ever before, present. They seem extra interested in suggesting medications than treating as well as preventing illness in a much more natural and also effective means. This is particularly perplexing as a growing number of people deal with wheat sensitivity, allergy, or celiac illness.

The problem with wheat is triggered by gluten, among the proteins located in modern-day wheat. It can harm the smaller intestine and make absorbing wheat tough or impossible. It can cause exhaustion, nausea, looseness of the bowels and various other, extra major pains, such as harming the small intestine. Celiac illness is severe, and also doctors require to begin focusing.

Processed wheat, which is discovered everywhere, isn't healthy and balanced for any individual. For people with celiac disease, it can be a daily problem. That is why going gluten-free is coming to be increasingly prominent. People are discovering the results of modern wheat and are beginning to take control of their own health and wellness.

For individuals who are sensitive or allergic to wheat, going gluten-free can be life-altering. It can help them free the body of bothersome toxins and help them work normally again.

For others, who are not gluten-sensitive, avoiding gluten is a way of eating much healthier, feeling much better, as well as having more energy.

Food issues. What we consume is essential to our health. The truth is, gluten includes little to our lives yet can create significant damage. Going gluten-free is a return to consuming in such a way that advertises maximum wellness as well as wellbeing. For any individual that thinks that we have actually been eating wheat for countless years without an issue, you will certainly quickly find out why that is incorrect.

Also for those who are not dealing with celiac illness or wheat level of sensitivity, a gluten-free diet can be an avoidance versus disease.

Gluten is recognized to cause serious swellings, and swellings can boost the risk of joint inflammation and coronary diseases. Using food to prevent the start of these problems enables us to enjoy a healthier way of living. This makes much more sense than treating diseases with medications that can have damaging adverse effects.

Gluten is throughout us, which can make going gluten-free fairly an obstacle. With numerous food items made from wheat, barley, or rye, every one of which include gluten, as well as with even more food consisting of concealed wheat, the idea of consuming gluten-free might appear like deprival. Quite the contrary. You can still eat the cookies, cakes, as well as pasta you like. You will just be preparing them differently.

If you are dealing with celiac condition, going gluten-free is a must. However various other intestinal problems, such as looseness of the bowels and also short-tempered bowel disorder have also been relieved with a gluten-free diet. Researchers are linking more and more gastrointestinal problems to gluten.

In addition, we'll take a look at the surprising connection between gluten-free, ADHD, and autism.

You will soon discover the options available to you, and how to make gluten-free eating a part of your healthy lifestyle.

CHAPTER 1

The Downside of Gluten

Wheat has been around for countless years. It's simple to grow and quite healthy. It was most likely one of the very first food items our predecessors collected to feed themselves. Wheat was genuinely lifegiving.

For all these countless years, the whole grain kernel was ground and used to bake bread or prepare cereals. Fresh, entire grain has always belonged of our diet plan without being damaging to our health.

It's not till the 1960s and 70s that people started to realize that the wheat they are taking in is making them sick.

What took place? Have our bodies altered? No. It's the wheat we have actually depended on for countless years that has been changed and twisted into something our forefathers wouldn't acknowledge.

Industrialization has actually been good to mankind, but it hasn't constantly respected the food we take in.

Let's begin with white flour, the very first food that we would call "processed." In 1870, the steel roller mill enabled wheat to be separated to fine-tune the wheat into a white powder. "White" flour was considered elegant.

So, to fulfill consumer demand, white flour was produced en masse, and the rest of the kernel, the healthy part, was tossed aside. Within ten years, all flour was white and seriously lacking in nutrients. 10 years was all the time it required to alter thousands of years of nourishment into something "elegant" and lacking in many nutrients.

That was only the beginning, nevertheless. By the 1950s, technology once again let us "enhance" our wheat. New methods allowed for genetically-altered seeds, fertilizers, and hazardous pesticides to increase wheat production. Again, everyone rejoiced. More wheat for everybody! Cake for one and all!

While the production of wheat increased, its dietary worth was being mangled into something indistinguishable. At the same time, swellings and immune illness were being linked directly to this brand-new, "enhanced" wheat.

Anybody who believes that gluten-free is just a modern stage is halfright. It is undoubtedly something new and modern. But it is not a phase. An increasing variety of individuals are struggling with the results of modern-day wheat and improved flour.

The degree can vary-- from a little wheat level of sensitivity to greater intolerance to celiac disease, which is the failure to process any amount of wheat due to issues in the small intestines. Particularly in the case of celiac disease, the digestive system views gluten as intruders and reacts appropriately. As it attempts to assault these toxins, the lining of the gut itself can become damaged, leading to leaks, inflammation, and other issues. Severe intestinal problems are the outcome.

The variety of individuals diagnosed with celiac disease has actually quadrupled in the past 50 years. One percent of the population experiences celiac illness, and the number is increasing. Wheat level of sensitivity affects approximately 8 percent of the population. It is obvious that new "improved" wheat is making people ill.

In studies comparing modern-day, "improved" wheat to old wheat (called Einkorn), it was discovered that the old wheat had no damaging impacts at all. No one who consumed unrefined wheat suffered any ill negative effects or gastrointestinal problems. The same studies showed that contemporary wheat can impact our autoimmune system in hazardous methods, resulting in celiac disease and allergic reactions.

Individuals who are not adverse modern-day wheat can still suffer. A 2013 study had healthy individuals consume either new or old wheat for 2 months. The group that consumed the old wheat discovered their cholesterol level had decreased and their level of potassium and magnesium had increased. The opposite held true of the group provided new wheat.

It is very important to compare gluten sensitivity and celiac illness, although they can have the exact same signs. Gluten level of sensitivity leads to feelings of fatigue, bloating, diarrhea, queasiness, and headaches. Many people don't even associate those feeling with wheat, so it's critical that physicians ask the ideal concerns and test for wheat allergy.

Individuals diagnosed with celiac disease suffer from identical signs, but the problem is more specifically specified. The gluten attacks the inflammatory system and can damage the small intestine. Swelling is related to a myriad of issues, such as heart disease, Alzheimer's, diabetes, and others.

The function of gluten itself is still being studied. What is clear, however, is that this modern-day, better wheat is causing some major disease. While wheat can be found practically all over, it is most frequently utilized in breads, cakes, cookies, pasta, creamed soups, sauces, cereal, and some salad dressings.

Rye wheat can be found in rye breads, beer, and some cereals.

Obviously, wheat can be discovered in many other hidden places, and we will discuss this in much higher detail.

What is clear is that individuals who have actually removed wheat and gluten from their diet plan feel better and end up being healthier. With anybody struggling with celiac illness going gluten-free is a requirement. For others, it is a choice in an effort to delight in increased health.

Many people also chose a gluten-free diet plan in order to slim down. A diet filled with breads, cakes, and noodles is high in carbs and will most likely pack on the pounds. The reason for that is that fine-tuned wheat can trigger a sugar spike. That indicates you use sugar for fuel while fat just gets stored and accumulated. People find reducing weight by cutting refined flour to be much easier and quicker.

Celiac disease can run in households and can be genetic. Individuals with parents or grandparents who have actually struggled with celiac disease have a 1 in 10 possibility of becoming grain-intolerant.

CHAPTER 2

Shopping Gluten-Free

When you begin to shop gluten-free, it can be a bit complicated and overwhelming. You might stress about missing out on your favorite meals. It may seem that there is absolutely nothing for you to consume. You'll rapidly discover, however, that is not the case. You won't miss anything.

Finding delicious foods that are gluten-free is easier than you believe. You are likely to discover a couple of delicious food choices that you have not thought about. Once you understand what to watch out for, you'll master the supermarket aisle like a gluten pro.

Besides, if several member of your household is gluten-intolerant while the rest are able to eat wheat, don't prepare separate meals. Gluten-free meals are NOT a penalty, and anybody suffering from celiac disease or gluten intolerance should not be made to feel guilty or various. Leaving out gluten from your diet is eating healthy, and that is something your entire family ought to be doing.

Have a Plan

Your trip to the market begins with a list. Pacing the aisles can cause serious temptations. Supermarkets are deliberately developed to tempt you and lure you into buying things you don't need. You do not want to wander arbitrarily. Before you leave your home, before you even create your shopping list, plan your meals.

Do not approach meal-planning adversely, as in, "Oh, I can't consume pasta ... bread ... cookies." Eating gluten-free is not about subtracting and deprivation. It's everything about consuming better. Strategy the meals you delight in and believe in terms of replacements. How can you improve this dish? For instance, if you want to prepare pasta, do so. Merely intend on using zoodles (zucchini noodles) or gluten-free pasta in your preparation.

Feel like baking some cookies for the kids? All you need to do is replace wheat-free flour in your recipe. We'll discuss substitution later in this book. One or two gluten-free cookbooks will provide you with motivation and help you comprehend how tasty gluten-free meals can be. They are an excellent financial investment.

Think in regards to range. The greater the range of food you eat, the more nutrition you consume. And do not ignore herbs and spices, the majority of which are rather nutrient-packed. Shopping gluten free will broaden your food world.

There are numerous locations to buy gluten-free products. (Aren't you fortunate!). There are the around-every-corner supermarkets, specialized shops, natural food stores, outside farmer markets, and online. By all means, make yourself readily available to all of these alternatives. Nevertheless, make the grocery store your main shopping location. There are factors for that.

First, gluten-free is catching on, and the majority of markets now bring gluten-free items or have an entire gluten-free aisle. The deli section is most likely to use a number of gluten-free items.

By shopping at the regular market, you will not feel that you are shopping "in a different way," which is mentally important. You're not different, you're simply smart.

Any farmer's market, naturally, is a treasure trove of healthy fruit and vegetables, so you definitely wish to be there whenever possible. When it comes to specialized organic food shops and online shopping, keep that in reserve as an important last hope for any product you can't find in stores.

Now that you have actually planed your meals, you are ready to produce your wish list. Remember that prepared and pre-packaged foods often have concealed sugars and gluten. If you are unsure, get in touch with the maker for more information. In addition to bringing your shopping list, you ought to also have a gluten-free food/ingredient list for translating tough labels.

We advise that if possible, you go shopping without kids, whose sticky little fingers inevitably grab chocolate, cookies, and other snacks with desert. You need to preserve control of the shopping scenario.

You at the Grocery store

Okay, you are at the supermarket, wheeling that shopping cart down the aisle. Now, what?

All supermarkets tend to be set out in the same way, so it's simple to avoid "harmful" aisles and sections. When shopping gluten-free, you'll be investing most of your time circling the perimeter of the store, and not the aisles.

The fruit and vegetables section is typically near the entrance, so that's where you want to head initially. Stock up on fresh, in-season vegetables and fruits. This is a chance to pick up produce you have not tried prior to and expand your food choice. Salads are constantly healthy, tasty, and gluten-free, but make sure with croutons and dressing.

The bread aisle can be challenging and appealing. You need to bypass a lot of bread offerings and search for gluten-free bread. Nevertheless, even here you require to be cautious. Anything labeled "gluten-free" may be filled with extra fats and sugars. In addition to studying labels carefully, take down the expiration date. Gluten-free breads normally have less preservatives and might expire quicker.

You have actually made it to the deli. You feel quite safe here, as cheeses do not consist of gluten. Technically, they do not, but numerous low-fat cheeses may include fillers that are wheat-based. As for cold-cut, they are most likely to contain wheat-based fillers. More about that later on, however ask the person behind the counter prior to making any purchases.

You must be able to make good use of the bulk food section. The bright side is there are numerous kinds of gluten-free, wheat-free flours from which to select. Gluten-free flours can function and taste in a different way from routine flours, so you need to end up being knowledgeable about how these flours are best used. A gluten-free cookbook can be very helpful in helping you create the scrumptious desserts you believed you 'd never ever take pleasure in once again.

A few of the most popular, gluten-free, wheat-free flours are as follows:

1. Coconut flour-- a terrific baking flour

2. Corn flour-- made from corn and utilized in baking and coating.

3. Oat flour-- when made from natural oats, oat flour is gluten-free. Great for cookies and baking.

4. Wild rice flour-- this is simple to absorb. In addition, pasta made with wild rice flour is your finest option to the standard white-flour pasta. There is white rice flour, also, which is gluten-free. Nevertheless, the white type of rice flour has actually been polished of the majority of its vitamins B and important minerals. It won't damage you, however you won't get the very same nutrition that you would with wild rice flour.

5. Almond flour-- made from healthy nuts. Almond flour can be used in nearly any type of baking.

6. Tapioca flour-- this isn't truly a baking/cooking flour. It is often utilized as a thickener for sauces and to develop a roux.

7. Chickpea flour-- this healthy flour consists of needed fiber and minerals. It is best utilized for pancakes and waffles.

8. Sorghum flour-- this is a heavy flour. When used in baking, it is regularly combined with tapioca flour.

9. Cassava flour-- this flour includes couple of nutrients aside from vitamin C, but it can easily be utilized for baking.

10. Amaranth Flour-- this is a nutrient-packed flour that, like sorghum, can be combined with another flour for baking.

11. Buckwheat flour actually isn't a flour, however a really healthful seed. Great for making pancakes.

12. Teff flour-- another flour that can be utilized with other gluten-free flours for baking.

13. Cricket flour-- this is actually made from roasted crickets, but don't let that keep you from trying it. It's nutrient-dense and has a nutty flavor.

14. All-purpose gluten-free flour-- this is made from a mix of the above flours and can be utilized for versatile baking.

As you can see, gluten-free cooking provides you lots of choices, and you ought to experiment to see which flour works best for you. Flours made from coconut or almond can provide a delightful taste to your baked items.

A word of care: When flours are shown wholesale, there can be some cross-contamination when a consumer uses the same scooper to bag glutenous and non-gluten types of flours. If that is a major concern, get your gluten-free flour from a market or a natural food shop that has a different gluten-free area, or order through the internet.

You and your cart, which is getting quite complete, have actually made it to the dairy section. Notice that you are still wandering the perimeter of the marketplace instead of roaming the aisles.

Milk and dairy do not contain gluten, however take care of ingredients. Yogurts and ice cream can consist of all types of flavoring, so read the labels thoroughly. And, as previously mentioned, any item identified "diet" or "slim" is most likely to include gluten fillers.

If you remain in search of treats, you are likely to end up in one of the aisles. Check ingredient labels carefully. As an option, prepare your own tasty snack by mixing gluten-free granola with chopped nuts or dried fruits.

When you arrive at the meat and fish section, you remain in a gluten free zone, except for the ready and coated meats, which you will disregard. Concentrate on lean meats and fish to prepare yummy and healthier meals.

CHAPTER 3

*Getting Started with the
Gluten-Free Life*

If you are thinking of going gluten-free in order to live more healthfully, great for you. It's an outstanding choice. If you have actually been diagnosed as gluten-intolerant, or even worse, with celiac illness, you might feel frustrated and overwhelmed. Where in the world do you even start? You have a right to be worried, since your health is at stake. Going gluten-free is a need to for you. It's up to you to make the experience as pleasurable as possible.

Your first step is to become as notified as you can, and the function of this book is to assist you begin. This is simply the start, nevertheless. Talk with a medical professional who is experienced and proactive when it pertains to diet plans and health; i.e., a medical professional who doesn't simply draw up prescriptions.

Consult with an experienced nutritional expert who recognizes with celiac illness. He or she can offer a great deal of in-depth information concerning your particular situation and assist you prepare healthy meals for you and your household. Then take a look at celiac support system in your location. Members have experienced the same frustrations you are now going through and will comprehend.

You also need to end up being product-savvy. Wheat can hide in the most unexpected places, especially in prepared foods. Read labels, and if you have any concerns, call the company and ask for specifics about the components. You have every right to understand what goes into your body.

A Gluten-Free Kitchen

As soon as you understand what foods to bring into your home (remember fresh is constantly best), you require to prepare your kitchen in order to avoid cross-contamination.

We have currently mentioned that it is best for the whole household to delight in gluten-free cooking instead of you preparing a separate meal. In the event you don't do that, you require to devote special home products to your gluten-free cooking. That includes pots, pans, cutting board, and utensils. Clean out the toaster to get rid of wheat crumbs. Gluten can attach itself to these products and cause cross-contamination.

Start your gluten-free journey from scratch. If the whole household is included, as they ought to be, throw out any gluten-containing food items from the freezer, refrigerator and cupboards and change them with gluten-free equivalents. It might appear frustrating to toss your preferred bagel, pasta, and cookies, once you learn how to prepare gluten-free alternatives, you won't miss them. There is every opportunity you will actual choose the delicious gluten-free meals and treats.

If other family members stay on a gluten-filled diet, position their food in a different, devoted location. After preparing their meals, be sure to thoroughly clean any afflicted surfaces.

Clearing out the Restroom

For anyone beginning on the gluten-free life, it may come as a surprise that the kitchen isn't the only room in the house filled with prospective risks.

Your bathroom might be equipped with gluten that can negatively affect your gluten intolerance. Numerous common cosmetics and hygiene items contain wheat. As a matter of fact, wheat is a favorite exfoliant for the face and body and can be discovered in any variety of creams and cleansers.

Check out the labels on the following bathroom items thoroughly:

- Soaps and gels

- Facial scrubs

- Hair shampoo.

- Skin creams.

- Tooth paste.

- Lipstick.

- Hairspray.

Much of these products call themselves "natural" or "organic" due to the wheat content. If you need to replace any item, search for products containing shea butter or oils such as coconuts or jojoba oil, which are outstanding moisturizers.

Fortunately, there are a number of cosmetic lines that specialize in gluten-free products. Inspect the internet for specifics.

In addition, if you are wheat-intolerant, beware of kissing somebody wearing lipstick that might include wheat. Guideline: if you understand someone all right to kiss, you should know them well enough to discuss your wheat-intolerance and have them examine their cosmetics.

You and Alcohol.

Fortunately is, you do not have to give up alcohol to delight in a gluten-free life. You do need to be careful of beer, distilled products, and any malt drinks.

You can, nevertheless, take pleasure in bourbon, gin, tequila, rum, cognacs, vodka, and red wine.

Gluten and Your Medication Cabinet.

While there is no remedy for celiac illness, you may be taking medications for other problems. While you can discuss medications with your physician, doctors aren't always informed about specific medicines and their active ingredients. Your best bet is to talk with the pharmacist and discuss your situation. It is constantly better to be informed and cautious.

A variety of pharmaceuticals consist of starch from corn, potato and wheat. Laws concerning labeling pharmaceuticals can be hazy. Companies are not required to note the kind of starch they use. Best to err on the side of care, as the incorrect medication may trigger abdominal problems, diarrhea and other symptoms. You do not desire your pharmaceuticals to make you sick!

If you have any doubts about the medication you are taking, have the pharmacist call the maker, or call the business yourself.

You are entitled to know how their items are produced.

While you're with your helpful pharmacist, ask him or her about supplements and vitamins. Given that celiac disease makes absorption of nutrients difficult (more about that in another chapter of this book), you need to be taking supplements to make up for the loss and aid alleviate nutrient shortage.

Gluten-Free Kitchen.

When you're consuming gluten-free, it is necessary to have a well-stocked kitchen. Otherwise, unforeseen visitors or getting home starving and wanting supper now, or simple, human cravings can have you throwing up your hands in anguish. "Fine, we'll purchase in pizza!".

If you do not desire that to occur, you need to be prepared with a well-stocked kitchen. You ought to have all the active ingredients for a delicious, gluten-free meal on hand whenever required.

Everybody turn to food for comfort sometimes. That's fine, as long as the comfort is healthful and nourishing.

For a quick breakfast when you remain in a hurry, keep a container of gluten-free buckwheat on hand. Try it with a poached egg to get your going in the early morning.

Have gluten-free breads on hand for a gratifying sandwich at lunch.

For a delicious dinner, make certain you have lots of gluten-free flours, brown rice, gluten-free corn tortillas to prepare meat and vegetable meals. Check out gluten-free pastas online.

Snacks can be difficult. When kids get back from school and bring their good friends, you need a plan. Be prepared to dish out popcorn, gluten-free crackers and cheese, trail mix, or banana slices with peanut butter at a minute's notice.

Essential Foods in Your Kitchen.

In addition to fresh produce and lean meats and fish, there are specific items that need to constantly be on your shelves. You will note that much of them are for spices and raising a meal when cooking. You actually must never be without:

- Garlic.

- Rice, quinoa and potatoes.

- Various kinds of gluten-free flours.

- A high-quality olive oil and other oils, such as coconut oil.

- A couple of high-quality vinegars.

- A range of lentils and bean, preferably the dry kind.

- A variety of broths, such as beef, chicken, and fish broths, preferably homemade.

- A range of nuts and seeds.

- Mustard.

- A range of spices to spruce up your dishes.

- Fresh herbs.

- Tamari sauce (a gluten-free soy sauce).

- Sour cream.

- Parmesan cheese.

- Eggs.

- Yogurts (check out labels prior to purchasing).

- Cans of tuna fish.

- Dried mushrooms.

- Canned tomatoes (check label).

- Fire-roasted tomatoes and chilis for added heat.

There are many other foods that can make it into your kitchen area, however these essentials ought to enable you to prepare a healthful, gluten-free meal at any time.

CHAPTER 4

At times, it might feel as if altering your consuming routines to get rid of gluten from your life is the worst thing that can take place. But then, as you find a world of healthy options and start to consume foods you have actually never ever even thought about, you unwind and delight in all the benefits.

There is one element of going gluten-free, however, that can unnerve even skilled old-timers. Eating someplace that isn't home. Managing eating in restaurants, either by yourself or with friends, can feel overwhelming. And how do you handle supper invitations? The fact is, other individuals may not comprehend what you are going through.

Unless you want to develop into a hermit, nevertheless, you are going to need to socialize. We are social beings, and we need to be around other people.

This book will assist you overcome the difficulties of eating out and turn you into a stress-free social butterfly.

Initially, you should not expect other individuals to accommodate your lifestyle. Some may be unaware, others might simply not know what to do and innocently prepare a meal they think you can consume. Comprehend that it's your duty, any place you are, to stay with your gluten-free diet. You can not, and shouldn't, rely on others.

What's For Supper?

It is rude to tell your host or hostess that you can't eat the lasagna which they should have something else for you. Do not anticipate unique accommodations. However, it is perfectly acceptable to just ask what they are serving.

Pleasantly explain that the factor for your query is that you have a dietary limitation. Perhaps the host will accommodate you; possibly not. However knowing what you're getting yourself into will assist you be prepared. You can eat prior to leaving for the event and then simply toy with a couple of veggies without calling attention to yourself.

What if your host guaranteed to prepare a gluten-free meal, but it ends up he or she has no concept what this involves and you end up with a fried chicken coated in flour? Again, it's a great idea to eat before getting here, in spite of the host's guarantees. Then, when you join the assembled visitors, you can concentrate on having fun instead of concentrating on the food. And don't sulk at the host. She or he indicated well however didn't understand much better than to serve anything breaded.

If you understand the host well, or if it's household, ask if you can bring your own dish that will accommodate your diet plan. Very few individuals would take offense to such a demand.

There will be times when neither you nor the host have enough control of the menu, such as when it's a big, catered affair. In such an occasion, do not even discuss your diet plan. Fill up on healthy food prior to you arrive. There is every possibility that such a function will have vegetables, salad, or a piece of meat that you can delight in. If in doubt, silently ask the catering staff.

As you go gluten-free, shift your mingling to having a good time with people instead of concentrating on the food.

You have actually Met Mr. or Ms. Right

Can you date and stay gluten-free? Of course, you can. It can be daunting until you get used to it, however if anyone carries on, she or he should have to be kicked to the curb, anyway.

A lot of first dates involve some type of food, so be upfront. Discuss that your food choices are limited due to health condition. How much you want to elaborate is up to you.

Offer to assist your date discover an appropriate restaurant. (" Billy-Bob's All You Can Consume Pizza" probably will not make the list.) If he or she opts to make the selection, you must feel free to get the name of the dining establishment ahead of time. Call the dining establishment prior to you go and inquire how they deal with gluten-free recipes.

A lot of dining establishments nowadays are willing to cooperate, but you want to make certain they don't cross-contaminate their ingredients. Ask how the food is prepared. These are not disrespectful questions, and any restaurant that treats them as such should not get your service.

If Mr. or Ms. Right minimizes your precautions, perhaps you ought to think about leaving them in the frog pond. Watching out for one's health is reasonable and wise.

At the restaurant, as you would in any social situation, concentrate on the other individual and have fun. The focus needs to be to enjoy, not worrying about the food. However do feel free to ask the waiter any pertinent concerns.

You're the Host

Most likely the best method to mingle and keep control of your diet plan is for you to be the host. This will not just relieve your concerns, it's a great chance for you to educate your loved ones.

When they inquire about a meal they take pleasure in, tell them it is gluten-free.

This is likely to promote their interest and raise questions about the advantages of eating gluten-free. Use this time to enlighten and inform your good friends. Who understands? You might make a few converts.

Discovering a Dining establishment

We have gone over calling restaurants and asking proper questions. Luckily, the number of gluten-free dining establishments is on the rise. When it comes to "regular" dining establishments, your best choice is one with a large and varied menu that will always have a simple steak and steamed veggies.

Specific types of dining establishments are most likely to be much safer for you than others.

1. BBQ restaurants are most likely to focus on meat and potatoes. BBQ sauces are typically gluten-free, but don't be reluctant to ask.

2. Do not discount junk food restaurants. The good thing about them is that they publish the nutritional content of all of their food. Fries, a salad, or some chili must be safe to consume.

3. Oriental restaurants such as Indian, Thai, or Vietnamese have rice noodles as a basic part of their menu.

4. Steak and Seafood restaurants are another good bet. Meat, fish, potatoes and a vegetable can make an exceptional gluten-free meal.

Simply stay away from anything breaded.

Make Gluten-Free Pals

If you sign up with a gluten-free support group in your area, you will satisfy brand-new people and make brand-new friends that are in the same position as you. You will be surrounded by an entire group that is encouraging and well-informed about gluten-free eating. That makes eating out and interacting socially a worry-free enjoyment.

CHAPTER 5

Preventing the Pitfalls of Gluten-Free

It's not just individuals with celiac disease that are choosing a gluten free diet plan. According to the Mayo Clinic, 72 percent of people going gluten-free are doing so on the recommendation of a nutritional expert or doctor. Thankfully, the medical occupation is no longer ignoring the fact that "new" processed wheat has absolutely nothing to offer us in terms of health and health and wellbeing and might be doing a variety of harm.

But getting on the gluten-free bandwagon without enough facts can backfire. Unless you make the effort to become informed, you are most likely to continue feeling not in addition to you could. The more you understand about gluten, where it is and what it does, the much better off you will be. The gluten-free life can be a challenge, and understanding is your best ally. If your small intestine is damaged, even small errors can cause a setback and prevent recovery.

One of the major obstacles is that gluten can hide in the most unanticipated locations. Going gluten-free is not simply a matter of abstaining from wheat products. Carefully read labels or ask concerns, since gluten may discover its way in the following food products:

1. Granola is hyped as an organic food, but many of them are made of glutenous oats. Read the label first.

2. Particular kinds of potatoes chips have malt (wheat) vinegar in them.

3. Meat is gluten-free, however beware of processed meats such as deli meats, hot dogs, salami, and liverwurst, as they are processed with grain.

4. Canned soups can contain barley or wheat as a thickening agent.

Again, read all labels.

5. Corn tortillas are typically gluten-free, but some add wheat.

6. Check all salad dressings and marinades.

7. Certain vegetarian "meats," such as vegetarian burgers, sausage or bacon, may contain gluten.

8. Some restaurants "puff" up their rushed eggs with wheat batter. If in doubt, ask the waiter.

In addition to the surprise gluten, another issue with developing a gluten-free diet plan is that you may not be getting all of the essential nutrients. According to a research study released in Medical Nutrition, gluten-free eaters were most likely to be lacking in vitamins D and B, zinc, magnesium, folate, iron and calcium.

The deficiency increases if non-glutenous bread, pasta, and so on are replaced for glutenous versions of these items. While gluten free foods can be practical and useful, a number of them are processed with added sugars and fats, and they are not "fortified" with extra vitamins the method white flour foods often are.

Gluten-free versions of any food will not make you ill, but you need to be very cautious.

Ensuring a nutrient-dense life is easy at all. Increase veggie and fruit portions to five a day and add quinoa and amaranth flour to your diet plan. The added vegetables and fruits will likewise provide you with the fiber you need.

To ensure that you get all your vitamins and minerals, consume a lot of the following foods:

1. Beas, peas, and vegetables are an exceptional source of thiamin.

2. Spinach and soybeans supply riboflavin

3. Avocado, chicken, broccoli, and salmon consist of niacin.

4. Greens, spinach, asparagus, broccoli, and lettuce give folate and magnesium.

5. For included iron, consume meat and lentils.

6. Seafood, specifically salmon, offers Vitamin D.

Celiac disease, which can harm the small intestine, can make it hard for the body to absorb all of the essential nutrients. Discuss taking a supplement with your doctor or pharmacist. To get all possible nutrients from the food you consume, increase your consumption of raw fruits and vegetables rather than cooking them. Choose a wide variety of produce that consist of as lots of colors as possible.

Another factor you may not be seeing the hoped-for progress on your gluten-free diet is that the damage to the small intestine is so extreme, even allowed grains such as rice or corn might continue to be a problem. Nuts, while gluten-free, are likewise tough to digest. If you continue to experience gastrointestinal problems, consult your doctor.

You may want to wait until your small intestine has actually recovered sufficiently before taking pleasure in those food products. Try to avoid all grains and nuts, even the permitted kinds, till your small intestine is back on track. This may take a while, so be patient. You desire the intestine to heal, don't you?

In addition, while gluten-free items can be practical, too many business are jumping on the gluten-free pattern. A lot of these items are over-processed and filled with sugars and fats and may come close to resembling any other processed food item. A better option is to buy a few respectable gluten-free cookbooks and prepare your meals from scratch.

Traveling Gluten-Free

You do not desire extra drama while taking a trip, however how are you expected to control your diet plan while on the road? Lots of people on a gluten-free diet plan unwind their eating habits due to poor planning.

As constantly, preparation is the crucial to success.

If you are driving, it's finest to prevent those roadside dining establishments. Merely pack a cooler with sandwiches on gluten-free bread. For snacks and for the kids, make certain you have lots of nuts, cheese, fruits (including dried fruits), and gluten-free crackers. Load the very same foods for flight travel and long waits at the airport. You can buy most type of potato chips securely (exempt malt vinegar flavored) at any airport newsstand.

Do some research study for any gluten-free restaurants along your travel route.

CHAPTER 6

*Emotional Obstacles to Having
Celiac Illness*

A diagnosis of celiac illness can appear frustrating. It's completely alright to feel upset. Celiac disease is serious, and it needs to be dealt with. You will unquestionably feel shock at the diagnosis. Your first response may be denial.

This can't be taking place to you! All you can feel is a squashing aggravation and anger at the unfairness of it all. These are perfectly typical responses. There is no reason for you to deny your emotions. Feel whatever you need to feel. After all, this medical diagnosis will alter a large part of your life.

At some time, you require to reach acceptance. You've been feeling sick and unpleasant for so long, you want to feel better. This is your chance. So, it up to you to end up being determined and handle the scenario.

Make no mistake. This may not be simple, especially if the decision to go gluten-free isn't your own. Here is why celiac disease can be such a hard medical diagnosis to accept:

1. Numerous of our social interactions revolve around food. You have every right to question how this will alter when you go glutenfree.

2. Family and friends may not understand your scenario. Perhaps a few of them tell you to just get over yourself. You may be accused of having an eating disorder. "It's simply toast and rushed eggs. Eat, for paradise sakes!" This lack of assistance just makes a difficult situation harder.

3. Knowing you'll need to give up a few of your favorite can produce reasonable anxiety. There is truth in the term "home cooking." Particular foods do comfort us. After your medical diagnosis, you realize your choices will be limited. You have certain favorite dishes that you might not have the ability to enjoy anymore. It seems like losing a pal.

4. You will require to make some modifications in your life. Depending upon how well you respond to change, that, too, can cause stress and anxiety.

5. You will have to follow brand-new rules, and that isn't always easy. You used to be in control of your consuming practices. Now you need to follow somebody's rules!

6. There is no recognized cure for celiac illness. All you can do is ease the symptoms by altering your eating habits. Yes, celiac is something you'll have to deal with forever.

7. Everybody around you is chomping on Oreo cookies and devouring hamburger buns. You feel alone and isolated.

8. A major issue for celiac patients is that they establish a gluten-free way of life, stick to it, and feel a lot better after a while. That's when the rumbling in the brain can begin. "I'm great now. I can have that piece of pizza or cookie." "Grandma prepared this specifically for me. I have to consume it." This can be among the most

tough periods you'll need to with. You're so lured ... simply one slice.

It's crucial to withstand temptation. You're feeling better due to the fact that you've eliminated gluten from your diet. Remember how unpleasant you felt before your new diet plan. Don't reverse the course that will require you to start over. You're exactly where you wish to be. Keep going.

When You Are Lured to Cheat

Often, the urge to cheat-- just a little bit-- can be frustrating. This is particularly true when special celebrations develop.

So many of our vacation memories are connected to food.

The problem is, there is no such thing as unfaithful "a little" when you have celiac illness. Even a minuscule amount of gluten can impact the immune system. So, it's not a matter of simply one bite." For someone with celiac illness, any bite is a bite a lot of. Even people who are "only" gluten-sensitive can be seriously affected by a small amount of it.

Gluten may trigger the gut to leak from the small intestine, which can cause contaminants to spread into the body and trigger inflammations.

Think about seriously if mommy's delicious stack of pancakes is worth this. This book is intended to assist you make great choices.

The most severe case of cheating is done by gluten-sensitive individuals who do not show immediate unfavorable signs. They might continue unfaithful, and gut is being damaged, although they do not understand it up until their autoimmune system is negatively impacted. If you have actually been exposed to gluten, get a laboratory test prior to the damage caused ended up being permanent.

Yearnings can appear at any time. They can be tough to handle, but you are in control. Like an alcoholic, take it one day at a time. You might desire that piece of cake more than life itself at this moment. Simply get through the moment. Leave, if possible. Understand that the yearning will not be as extreme the next day. We duplicate: manage cravings one day at a time and remain in control.

You also need to comprehend what foods trigger your cravings. Is it going to mom's house and having her prepare all of your youth favorites? Is going out with pals for pizza too difficult to handle?

If you can't prevent the triggers (you actually can't prevent mother), find out to manage them. Talk with mother about celiac illness and how to prepare gluten-free options; or bring your own. Discover pizza parlors with gluten-free choices and convince your good friends to go there. Keep in mind, unfaithful is constantly a choice. Make good choices on your own.

Taking Control of Your Emotions

Let's not deceive ourselves. Knowing you are experiencing celiac illness can cause bouts of blues and anxiety. When you start feeling down, it's time to raise your emotions instead of obsessing on food. Following are some ways to feel better and delight in a higher quality of life.

1. Depression can make you withdraw, but you need to connect. Have at least one person you can speak to about what you are going through without stressing over judgments being made.

This can be a parent, sibling, buddy, someone else who has celiac disease, or an expert. Simply feeling understood can lift your spirits significantly.

2. Instead of withdrawing, end up being more included with individuals. Reach out to someone who is going through a rough time. Find a beneficial association where you can volunteer and make a distinction. Everyone is dealing with something. Knowing that will make you feel less alone.

3. While a family pet will not change other individuals, it can help you feel less alone.

4. Discover a new hobby or interest to get your mind off food. Taking a class, joining a health club, becoming associated with your neighborhood can be very energizing. Life has too much to use to make it all about food.

5. If particular individuals are unsupportive of your situation or maybe really accusing you of overreacting, think about whether these people should remain in your life? Exactly what are they adding to it?

6. Remove as much stress from your life as possible. Think about practicing meditation for half an hour daily. Just find a comfy seat, close your eyes, and concentrate on your breath as you breathe in and breathe out. This will relax your mind and spirit.

7. Nature seems to be the best medicine of all. If you live in a city, find a park and walk around, enjoying what nature has to provide. Take a walk throughout your lunch hour. If you reside in the nation, communicating nature is even much easier. It holds true that sunlight will boost your day.

CHAPTER 7

Gluten, ADHD, and Autism

ADHD-- attention deficit disorder-- is on the increase. It is challenging to identify (and reward), however as the name indicates, it includes the amount of hyperactivity in children. The connection between celiac disease and ADHD is still being studied, but physicians and parents have actually discovered that both are connected to food allergic reactions and/or food intolerance. Interestingly, around 70 percent of ADHD patients have a sensitivity to gluten.

We know that the frontal brain lobe, which supervises of memory and preparation activity suffers in individuals with ADHD. It is also understood that gluten can affect that really area of the brain. Therefore, a growing number of scientists and medical professionals are dealing with ADHD by omitting gluten from the diet.

Kids with ADHD react differently when gluten is eliminated from their diet plan. However the results have been quite unbelievable. The kids have actually become less hyperactive and reduced mental confusion. In each study, the scientists discovered that quitting gluten led to enhanced brain function in all cases.

When the connection in between autism and gluten was studied, twothirds of the kids showed improvement once they were no longer eating gluten. They are still working to connect the two elements, but the outcomes have amazed them. They can not be denied.

One of the challenges for parents, naturally, is particular little eaters. Some kids are exceptionally adamant in what they will consume and what they won't go near. They may only eat one sort of food or perhaps food of one color. Kids with ADHD may also react adversely to sugar, so parents need to get rid of both from their diet.

In a 2006 research study, 132 participants were evaluated for celiac disease and ADHD. Consequently, the participants were provided a diet plan without gluten for 6 months. When the researchers inspected them after that time period, they found that numerous participants with undiagnosed celiac illness also had ADHD. They concluded that a diet plan free of gluten could benefit these individuals.

Both people struggling with celiac illness and ADHD reveal man.

Celiac disease sufferers complain of many comparable pains: signs as ADHD patients do. This might include headaches, problem in focusing, abdominal pain and others. Researchers have notice such an overlap in signs that some believe that anybody evaluated for celiac illness ought to instantly be screened for ADHD.

Naturally, not all people with ADHD suffer from celiac disease however may still gain from a gluten-free diet. The factor is that a gluten free diet plan, when effectively adhered to, ought to be more nutrient-dense than the average diet plan. This means that someone with ADHD on a gluten-free diet plan will be consuming less processed foods and consume more healthy meats, fish, and produce and see symptoms enhance as a result.

All-to-frequently, when kids with ADHD go to school, the gluten free diet is quit as unsustainable. These kids find it tough to sit still for lengthy time periods. This forces them back on medication. A variety of parents have actually solved the issues by reinstituting a gluten-free diet (yes, it's tough to control kids when they are in school). Parents have actually discovered that the kids enhanced enough to have their medication lowered substantially.

Gluten-Free and Autism

So far, there has actually been insufficient research on autism and gluten-free diet plans. Autism is a condition of the brain which can make it difficult for a kid to interact and mingle.

Stony Brook University researchers studied 59 children identified with autism and 44 of their non-autistic siblings. The children's family were to tape all of their food intake and take stool samples.

The scientists discovered that almost half of the autistic kids, and 30 percent of the non-autistic brother or sisters, struggled with gastrointestinal disorder. These numbers are much higher than found in the general population of children. Given that gastrointestinal issues included the small intestine, scientists have concluded that a gluten-free diet might show helpful.

If your child struggles with AHDH or autism, talk about the possibility of a gluten-free diet with his/her pediatrician. While more studies require to be carried out, positioning your kid on a healthy gluten-free diet won't harm him or her, and it may help. Be sure to go over any specific dietary modifications with your child's doctor.

Be careful of Chocolate

Kids love chocolate, and you do not wish to deny them. The bright side is, you and the kids do not need to give up your favorite sweet on your gluten-free diet plan. You simply have to pick the right chocolate bar. Some are gluten-free, others aren't.

The issue isn't chocolate, as the cacao bean is naturally gluten free. Nevertheless, a lot of sweet bars include a variety of active ingredients, and that's what you need to look out for. A general rule is that the more ingredients in a chocolate bar, the higher the chances there will be a wheat by-product.

Chocolate bars that contain a cookie are off-limits. Malt balls are made with malt and include gluten.

Milk chocolates such as Hershey's Milk Chocolate Bar is made with milk and is gluten-free.

When it comes to white chocolate, you need to check out the labels. Typically, white chocolate is made with sugar and shea butter and is gluten-free. But that does not apply to every brand name of white chocolate. Lindt's white chocolate contains gluten, while Ghirardelli's White Chocolate baking bar does not.

While many chocolate manufacturers make gluten-free chocolate, they use the same equipment to produce their gluten chocolates without cleaning the makers, thereby risking cross-contamination.

Chocolate-lovers can unwind, however. There are a number of safe, gluten-free chocolates on the market:

- Alter Eco-- almost all of their premium chocolates are gluten free.

- Nestlé Milk Chocolate is gluten-free

- Dove Chocolate-- these chocolates contain no gluten.

- Enjoy Life chocolate-- These chocolate bars are manufactured on gluten-free devices and are completely gluten-free.

- Hershey's-- The popular Hershey Kisses and the Hershey milk chocolate are gluten-free. Their other candies may include gluten.

- Scharffen Berger Chocolate makes both dark and milk chocolate bars that are gluten-free.

- Vosges Haut Chocolate makes chocolates with some interesting tastes, the majority of which are gluten-free. Inspect the label.

To keep your kid from being lured by chocolate when amongst good friends, tuck a couple of satisfying Hershey's Kisses in his or her bag.

CHAPTER 8

Adjusting Your Diet to Gluten-Free

Once you go gluten-free, you can still delight in the exact same dishes you have actually constantly liked. As currently stated, you aren't quiting anything; you are adding better health to your life. You just require to get imaginative about preparation methods. Keep in mind that almost any meal can be made gluten-free.

Baking Your Favorite Treats the Gluten-Free Way

We guaranteed at the beginning of this book that you could relish your preferred cookies, pies, and cakes on a gluten-free diet. Utilizing gluten-free flours can be difficult, however it's still possible to create delicious goodies on your own and your family. Here are some tips for altering your gluten-sweets into gluten-free:

1. When utilizing gluten-free flour, increase the baking powder and baking soda by a quarter. If a basic recipe calls for a teaspoon of baking soda, use a teaspoon and a quarter.

2.Gluten-free flour can fall apart. For that reason, making smaller sized variations of your usual cookies, or baking private pies instead of one big one, will assist keep everything stuck. When baking breads, bake 2 mini-loaves instead of a single loaf.

3. Enhance the quality and taste of baked goods by combining different types of gluten-free flour instead of using just one kind.

4. Use starches for added texture when you bake. Every recipe can vary, so you need to experiment. A great guide is to utilize 3 cups of flour to 1/2 cup of starch. Starch can be tapioca, potato starch, or cornstarch. It bears repeating that baking is not an accurate science, and you might need to experiment a couple of times with the ratio for the best mix.

5. Gluten is what assists a dough stick. Without gluten, you need to utilize something else to keep your meal from breaking down. Use a teaspoon or more of guar gum, gelatin, or xanthan to keep your breads together. For cakes and muffins, include just half a teaspoon. Including an additional egg can also assist bind the dry active ingredients together.

6. Yes, you are likely to make errors when you experiment. But you do not need to let whatever go to waste. Place those errors in a food mill and produce gluten-free covering for your fried meats and fish.

7. To develop a more ideal gluten-free dough, beat the batter more than you would regular dough to provide it with some structure.

8. Butter is an allowed addition to your gluten-free baking. Nevertheless, to include extra sweet taste, wetness, and nutrition, substitute a portion of the butter called for with a fruit puree. The very best fruits to use are apples, avocados, and bananas. They can add a good deal of taste to baked products.

Making Good Replacements in Your Recipes

Get creative when cooking gluten-free and learn how to multi-use your active ingredients:

1. Anything that calls for a bun can be wrapped in lettuce or a corn tortilla.

2. You do not need to quit your favorite fried chicken, pork chops, or fish. Just replace a different finishing for the typical breadcrumbs. We have already talked about turning some stopped working baking attempts into crumbs. You can likewise turn gluten-free bread into breadcrumbs. Another intriguing method to coat is to crumble up pork rinds.

3. Some recipes require beer. Unless you have a non-malt, gluten free beer handy, use apple cider rather.

4. To make croutons for your salads, cut up a couple of pieces of gluten free bread and fry the cubes.

5. When preparing sandwiches, don't limit yourself to gluten-free bread. Get imaginative and utilize corn tortillas, waffles, or thin pancakes. Likewise, attempt a healthy lettuce wrap.

Mastering gluten-free cooking takes some creativity and experimentation. It's an excellent idea to try smaller batches until you accomplish rewarding outcomes.

Being diagnosed with celiac disease or wheat allergy does not have to disrupt your preferred meals. Play around with the ingredients and delight in yummy outcomes.

CONCLUSION

Receiving a diagnosis of celiac illness or gluten intolerance can be a shock that can come out of the blue. Even if you've made your own choice to abstain from consuming gluten for reasons of health, you may feel rather overloaded. You understand modifications are needed, but how do you even get going?

Understand that quitting some of your favorite food items is a loss, particularly when you didn't anticipate it. Allow yourself time to feel that loss.

1. You want to reject what the doctor is telling you. She or he can't possibly be right. Medical professionals make mistakes all the time. While you remain in denial, nevertheless, you feel exhausted, uneasy, and continue reacting terribly to wheat.

2. You blow up. Who is somebody to inform you that you can't go to your preferred pizza place!

3. After you deal with the anger, you psychologically attempt to negotiate with yourself. OK, so I might have celiac disease. But eating just one breeze at the celebration can't perhaps injure.

4. When the fact sinks in, you are likely to feel depressed. My life is over!

5. It may take a while, however approval lastly embeds in. You do some research and recognize you can still eat what you want and do what you have actually always done. The only real modification in your life will be that you begin to feel a lot better than you have in the past.

When you have moved your mindset, you are ready to start going gluten-free. Once you understand the health advantages of giving up that unrefined flour, it is doubtful you will be seriously tempted to go back to the old, glutenous methods of eating. Going gluten-free is a lifetime commitment.

- Do some research study and find out how wheat has actually changed from a life-sustaining food staple to a mangled grain that lots of people can not process. The gluten in grain is in fact making individuals ill.

- Rid your home of all gluten. Clean out the pantry, fridge and examine the bathroom cabinets for any items consisting of gluten. Clean your pots, pans, and utensils to make sure that no cross-contamination occurs. Gluten can connect itself to lots of products in your home.

- Knowing how to browse the supermarket aisles when shopping will assist you stockpile on fresh, healthy food items and avoid harmful temptations. It is very important to always have a couple of staples on hand for fast meals and treats. This will keep you from reaching for something that can ultimately make you ill. Plan your meals before you go shopping to make certain you have the essential ingredients on hand.

- Even if you are removing gluten from your diet does not mean you can't continue interacting socially and eating in restaurants with family and friends. Many dining establishments nowadays have the ability to accommodate a gluten-free diet plan. Take a look at regional eateries and inquire about their cooking process.

When dining at the home of family and friends, don't anticipate them to change their eating routines for you. They might try, but they might not know what to do. If in doubt, eat something healthy prior to visiting and focus on delighting in the business. Don't be reluctant to discuss your dietary limitations when the subject emerges.

- If you start a gluten-free diet without understanding exactly what the diet requires, you could be undercutting your efforts. It's not just about eliminating breads, cookies, and cakes. Gluten can hide in numerous foods, so discover to read labels with great care. Make sure your diet plan isn't nutrient-deprived by consuming lots of fresh produce every day. Consume a wide range of foods to enjoy the best possible nutritional advantage.

- Even as you feel better and more energetic, you may still have moments of sensation denied. That is completely normal. Discover daily practices that let you deal successfully with unfavorable feelings. Including workout and new activities to your regimen will broaden your way of life and keep you from focusing only on food.

- Numerous intriguing studies are being done with gluten and kids with ADHD and autism. A lot more research is needed, but a variety of tests have actually revealed that eliminating gluten from the diet of children suffering from ADHD or autism has had an extremely useful impact. This is something that should be talked about with your child's pediatrician.

- Baking, which constantly entails utilizing flour, can be the most significant gluten-free difficulty. Learn about all the alternatives you can make to prepare your old preferred treats and the very best cooking methods for gluten-free baking. You will be happily shocked.

Celiac illness and wheat allergies hurt. If you are gluten sensitive, there is no reason for you to feel unpleasant. Take the essential steps to rid your life of gluten and start enjoying every day again. This could be one of the most important health choices you will ever make.